London Call-Out

LONDON CALL-OUT

Confessions of a Doctor in the Capital

ALEX RUDD

LUME BOOKS

LUME BOOKS

This edition published in 2021 by Lume Books
30 Great Guildford Street,
Borough, SE1 0HS

ISBN 978-1-83901-322-5

Typeset using Atomik ePublisher from Easypress Technologies

www.lumebooks.co.uk

Author's Note

I was thrilled when I was asked to write about life as an evening and night-time GP in London. I really hope people enjoy reading about it – and I apologise if sometimes my spelling, punctuation or my grammar can be as bad as my handwriting. I've been doing this job for a while so I've tried to cover a variety of different incidents, topics and opinions to give a real flavour of life in the small hours. Over the past few years I've really enjoyed books by the likes of Benjamin Daniels, Nick Edwards, Max Pemberton, Tom Reynolds, Ben MacFarlane, Rosemary Leonard and several other doctors. I've taken their cue and changed patient names, locations and other details to preserve everyone's confidentiality. What I've really tried to do, though, is to show that for all the criticisms, our NHS really does do its absolute best to look after us. It might take a while, but if you or your family need help in the middle of the night or at the weekend then you'll get it. Thanks for reading.

Chapter One:

The First Call

'Hello Doc, fancy a trip to deepest Hackney?'

It's just gone 3am in late February. It's warm and dry in my surgery and looks horribly wet and windy outside. I've just made myself a coffee and I've got a big backlog of phone calls to return. But it looks like I'm going to Hackney.

'This had better be good, Steve. I'll get my bag and see you in the car.'

Five minutes later I've downed one coffee and put a second one in a travel cup. I've logged off my computer, told the nurses I'm going on a house-call and headed out to the hospital car park. I'm wearing black cargo trousers, a dark blue jumper and a waterproof hiking jacket. I could probably pass for a burglar, an off-duty copper or a tourist with a bad case of insomnia. In fact I'm an out-of-hours doctor, part of a team of half a dozen or so GPs, nurse practitioners and drivers that takes over this set of empty rooms in a London medical centre from six in the evening till eight the following morning.

Steve is one of our drivers. At this particular centre they can be the first to know when one of the GPs needs to do a house-call. If they're hanging around by the phones and printers they'll find out who needs a doctor and where. They then walk down the corridor to see whether any of their favourites are free.

'So, where are we off to?' I ask Steve as we cut across some empty roads and head north. I was brought up in Blackburn so Steve knows London a lot better than I do. He used to be a black cab driver, he ran a private hire chauffeur service for a while and now he earns a decent amount driving doctors around four nights a week. He's always got an opinion or a story. Tonight is no exception.

'Last time I took someone up here it was the night after a riot. Looked like bleedin' Beirut. Bins in the road, police everywhere, whole gangs of idiots roaming around trying to karate-kick wing mirrors and acting like animals on bleedin' acid,' he tells me with relish. Rain is sweeping across the windscreen and the wind slams against the car as we wait at one particularly exposed red light. It looks like one of those nights when no one will hear you scream. In the olden days, GPs doing house calls were easy targets, especially in tough parts of town. We travelled on our own and low life reckoned we had plenty of juicy kit in our bags – prescription drugs and shiny kit and lots of other goodies you could use yourself or sell on the street. Medical school is full of tall tales of doctors lured to non-existent addresses and mugged for their medicines.

As it turns out, the address we're looking for tonight is in one of the more posh parts of Hackney. We leave the high-street fried chicken shops behind and drive through a set of increasingly attractive residential squares. I'm doing night shifts because I want to save up to move house. This is exactly the kind of area I'm aiming for. Most of the houses look well pointed, well painted and share a distinct lack of old mattresses or washing machines in the front gardens. If I get mugged here it's because someone wants my double espresso.

'That looks like the place,' Steve says as the sat-nav he doesn't need tells us we've reached our destination. The whole street is dark – except for one house that has light blazing from every window. Steve double parks outside, flicks on the hazard lights and tells me to have fun.

'Hello, I'm Doctor Rudd. You called for a GP.'

A man in his mid-forties has opened the door for me. He looks tired, worried and just a little bit beaten. He smiles, opens his mouth to say hello and steps back to let me in when a small, wild-haired woman pushes past him. Her eyes are flashing with anger. She's only about five-foot five but she's got momentum on her side. She forces her way out on to the garden path and I step back to give her some space. The rain hammers down as she squares up in front of me. This woman, it is clear, is up for a fight.

'You're not coming in. I told him not to call you,' she spits out.

'We've had a call about an elderly lady who's in some distress,' I begin. 'Is it your mother?'

'Yes it's my mother and it's nothing to do with you and it's nothing to do with him,' she says, firing a vicious glance back to the man in the hallway.

'She needs help, love,' he says very quietly. 'She's in a lot of pain and it's getting worse. She needs help.'

'I can look after her. She's my mother. '

'Shall I just take a look at your mother? What's her name?'

'What's it got to do with you? I know why you're here and I know what you want to do. You're going to take her back to hospital and I won't let you. I swear I won't let you in my house if you take her to hospital.'

I relax, just slightly. Now I understand. Now it's clear.

'How long has your mother been unwell?' I ask. 'Do you want to explain it to me inside, out of the rain? I don't need to see her straight away but I do need to see her.'

The woman almost sways with indecision. She looks as if she's going to raise her fists, then she drops them. She looks through me as she sweeps a handful of wet black hair away from her face and takes a big gulp of air. She looks so tired I wonder, for a moment, if she might fall. 'I won't let you take her to hospital,' she repeats, though her voice is quieter now.

'I'll do the very best I can for your mother. Let's go inside.'

It's a warm, pleasant house. I shake the rain off my coat and wish the carpet wasn't so pale. I sit on the edge of a vast red sofa in a sparse but stylish front room. Glossy framed magazine covers line the walls. 'She's sleeping now,' the woman tells me softly.

'She sleeps for about twenty minutes at a time,' says the man. 'But every time she wakes it's worse. Tonight's been worse than ever. That's why I called.'

'It's cancer,' the daughter says, answering my unspoken question. 'Pancreatic cancer. She'd not been well but she doesn't like doctors and refused to be looked at for far too long. She was only diagnosed four weeks ago. It's very, very late stage, I think. We moved her here as soon as we could. I thought I could look after her on my own but she's in so much pain. Sometimes she can't breathe. Tonight she's been worse than ever.'

'Is she upstairs?'

4

The woman nods but her eyes, and her mind, are elsewhere. 'I promised her I'd look after her,' she says. 'We've not always been close. I've not always been kind. So I have to do this now. I have to make things right on my own. I can't let her go back to hospital.'

'What's your name?'

'Julie.'

'Julie I can't know what will be best for your mother till I see her. And I have to see her.'

'She'll die on some ward. She says such terrible things about hospitals. I can't send her back to die on her own.' Julie is crying now, fat, single tears turning into streams as they pour down her face. She wipes them away and clutches her chest as if she, too, is finding it hard to breathe.

I stand up. It's time to move this along.

'I'll see your mother now,' I say firmly. Julie gives the tiniest of nods. She leads me upstairs.

The back bedroom is peaceful. It's calm. And it is very sad. Julie's mum looks like a very small doll on a very large bed. Her skin is far too big for her body. The weight must have fallen off her fast. In the soft light of the room you can make out far too many of the bones in her hands. She stirs and opens her eyes as I approach. They're a very pale blue. They fix on me as a shadow, then a frown, then a spasm of pain cracks across her forehead.

'What's your mum's name?'

'Pamela. Pamela Hany.'

'Hello Mrs Hany, Pamela. I'm Doctor Rudd. Don't try to move. I'm here to help you. Can you hear me OK?'

The spasms are strong and fast now. Pamela opens her mouth wide, gasping for air. Pain can hit you like a wave of ice cold water. The shock can go through to your core. The fear it brings can overwhelm you.

'Can't bear it. Can't bear it,' she whispers, forcing out the words from far away. Wishing, I imagine, that she was somewhere far away herself.

'It's OK, I can help you, just stay as calm as you can,' I say as I run through my initial checks and work out the lady's existing treatment schedule. Symptom control for the terminally ill is a big part of what we all do at night. We rarely re-invent the wheel on occasions like this. Unless we spot something that other people have missed it doesn't make sense to start people on new medications. Our primary role is to make people as comfortable as they can so they can get through to morning.

'I can increase the pain relief that your mother is getting,' I say, after listening very quickly to her chest to see if there's an infection or any extra fluid on her lungs. I'm stating a fact rather than asking for permission. But Julie seems to hold back from giving it, all the same. In the end her husband speaks.

'Please just do it,' he says firmly as I check the syringe driver at the lady's side.

The job is done in no time at all. I could provide something else for agitation but Mrs Hany is calm. She's suffering a lot less now. There is, though, a lot of tension between her daughter and her husband. It was right of him to face her down and call us out. But I'm not sure she sees it that way just yet.

Back on the landing Julie confirms how conflicted she is. She grabs my arm. She looks at the floor, the ceiling, and everywhere but at me. She takes a while to speak. 'Am I doing the right thing?' she asks in the end. There's even more desperation on her face. She still won't look me in the eye, but it is clear she has something to say. 'I'm not a fool. I'd hate it and my mother would hate it but if hospital can stop the pain then I will listen. You can take her now. I will let her go if it's kinder.'

I try to reassure her – and it's not hard because I agree with her. Certain categories of patients will need the full spectrum, 24-hour care you can only get in a hospital. But far too many older people end up parked in a noisy ward because once you're in you weaken so fast that you can't then be discharged. So many of these lost patients would be better off if they'd never been admitted in the first place. Pamela is one of them. She'll be more comfortable and more loved at home. She'll be less lonely, less isolated and a lot less likely to get MRSA. Throw that little horror into the mix and it's easy to understand the old joke about hospitals being some of the most dangerous places on earth.

Julie and I stand on the landing and talk for a short while about hospices, palliative and respite care and all the other logistics of looking after her mother at home. A lot of the incredible, unseen and unsung support that this country offers is already in place – though Julie admits she's been as unwelcoming to them as she was to me. She's had her own GP, district nurses, palliative care nurses and Macmillan nurses in the house – and every time they visit she says she panics and thinks they're going to take her mother away with them. 'All of them are here to help your mother and to help you. They'll listen to everyone's wishes, they'll explain everything and they'll do what's best. That's what all of us will do,' I tell her.

Julie looks at the floor. 'One of the first district nurses was really amazing,' she says very softly and very slowly. 'She was the one who put in the syringe thing. She helped so much and

I couldn't bring myself to speak to her. But she spoke to my children. She sat them down in the kitchen and she explained things better than I ever could. I didn't even thank her. I didn't even say goodbye when she left the house. I'm so ashamed of that.'

I put up my hand to interrupt her. 'Just thank her next time,' I say firmly. 'She'll appreciate it and she will understand.'

Julie nods, frowns and leads me slowly down the stairs. I pull my coat back on when she asks the question. It's the question doctors always dread.

'How long does she have?'

I don't know, of course, and I couldn't say even if I did. You never know how fast cancer will take someone. Strong people can fade fast while the weak can defy all the odds and carry on for months or even years. Instinct and experience tells me that Pamela will go soon, but I keep that entirely to myself. Julie accepts the non-committal answer I conjure up. Her husband thanks me for coming and says goodbye. Then she steps forward.

'I'm sorry I was so terrible before. I can't believe I shouted at you in the rain. It's the middle of the night and I can't believe I wouldn't let you inside,' she says. This time there's an embarrassed, unbelieving smile on her face. This, I imagine, is the real Julie.

'People have done a lot worse at this time in the morning,' I tell her. 'And my night's not over yet.'

Chapter Two:

Working Nights

Working nights isn't for everyone. Years ago it was part of every GP's job. That's why people hark back to the 'good old days' when they reckon their family GP was happy to leap on to his bicycle at 2am and cross town with a winning smile on his face if little Johnnie woke up with a sore throat. Not anymore. About ten years ago GPs were offered the chance to opt in to the system and earn lots of extra cash, or opt out and leave nights to someone else. Almost all of them opted out.

Ring your local surgery as little as one minute past its normal business hours and there's zero possibility that you'll speak to one of your usual receptionists. Instead your call will click on to an answerphone message and redirect you, or it will go through to a specialist out of hours or OOH company, a big regional call centre or one of the other constantly changing services that aims to give us a 24/7 health service.

Once those calls are answered the details come through to people like me – and in some parts of the country people like me are a bit thin on the ground. That's why doctors have been brought in from overseas at a vast cost and with varying results – but more of that later.

A lot of the doctors I trained with think I'm mad to be a locum and positively certifiable to do nights. But I really enjoy it. I prefer the phrase 'sessional GP' to locum. But either way it certainly beats sitting at the same desk seeing the same hard core of patients all the time. Doctor friends who work 'normal' hours are always moaning about writing sick notes for people who know how to fake a bad back, depression, stress or a genetic addiction to cake. They say they spend a huge chunk of their time reassuring the worried well. We can get a fair bit of that in the out-of-hours world as well. But we avoid all the office politics and we have a lot more variety. Things really do go bump in the night. I like picking up the pieces afterwards.

Evening, night-time or weekend out-of-hours shifts let you cover far more ground than a typical GP's practice. I work in several different centres across London and tonight my little team of six will cover for several different boroughs, dozens of surgeries and several hundred thousand patients. The total ground we cover probably spreads over some thirty-five square miles of the Capital. That said, even we get to see the same patients on a regular basis. They are the city's night-time frequent flyers. Some are in genuine need. Others play the system. They've long-since worked out the key words to tell the phone staff so their calls monkey up the triage system and trigger a home visit. As far as I know the set-ups vary around the country. In theory us GPs always have the final say and can approve or refuse a trip to someone's home. But in some out-of-hours services it's other people who read computer scripts and do what the latest NHS pathway tells them. Either way, the frequent flyers should get flagged up as such – and if they come into the surgery a note should pop up on the GP's screen with a bit of background.

So why do patients call up or come in so often? Loneliness is as big a factor as illness. Everyone needs a friend and a hobby. Sometimes a doctor is someone's only real friend, and a home visit or a trip to the surgery in the early hours is their one big hobby.

And why do the staff do it? Like I say, I work nights because the money is nice and I don't want to be ground down by routine. The company can be good as well. The faces change, but there's a hard core of late-night regulars in some of London's out-of-hours centres. The best centres are the smaller and more traditional set-ups. If we get a quiet patch in one of these co-operatives there's a real camaraderie between the doctors, nurses and drivers. That's normally down to people like Annie.

Annie has been a night nurse for about fifteen years. She's a tiny, firecracker of a woman. She's from Ghana, her husband is from Birmingham and she lives in Bermondsey. Her accent is all over the place. We bonded on one of my first night-shifts about five years ago. I'd been called to an old guy's house to change his catheter – and it turned out I wasn't alone. The district nurse had already been – and she'd not managed to do it. When I arrived another nurse was pitching up as well. That was Annie. 'They call me the Catheter Queen,' she said proudly as I tried to work out why so many of us had been given the same call-out.

She wasn't on very good form that night, though. The man we were helping hadn't been able to pee for hours and was in a whole lot of pain. Imagine your bladder so full to bursting that urine is backing right up into your kidneys. No one will be on good form when their bladder is the size of a water melon – and this man was clearly a cantankerous old sod at the best of times. 'Don't just ram it up there!' he howled, outraged, as Annie got her gloved hands on his nether regions and began the job. We put some anaesthetic lubricant and antiseptic in place then ease the tube through the man's urethra to his bladder. Or at least that's the idea. Tonight nothing seemed to be working. 'If you're the catheter queen you're a bit cack handed tonight,' I remember thinking to myself – sorry Annie. But she was certainly determined. She gave it another go, then another, and all the while pressure was building up for our poor patient.

'Let me have a go,' I said after another failed attempt. Call it beginners' luck but I got the tube where it needed to go straight away. After the final few twists the balloon end entered the man's bulging bladder, we made sure it was fixed in place, attached a drainage bag and the pressure – for me and my patient – was well and truly off. The waters began to flow and I doubt there was a happier man in London. That's one reason why staff quite like doing catheter jobs. It's a bit intimate and fiddly – but patients feel so good so fast that they'd probably give you their car if you asked. The night I met Annie, we regulated the flow a bit till the waters ran dry. Then we all gave deep sighs of relief. Our job was done.

'I did all the groundwork for you,' Annie declared with absolute certainty – and just the hint of a smile – as we packed up the used swabs, antiseptic and anaesthetic gels.

'Course you did,' I began – just as the lights went out.

'It's the fuse,' the old man's wife told us. A bulb in the hall had blown and tripped it. So five minutes later I was half way up a step-ladder by the front door, trying to repair an ancient fuse box in pitch black while the catheter queen stood by my feet holding the world's smallest and least effective pen torch.

'I bet I could have done the catheter in the dark as well,' I told Annie once we'd left.

'Only if I'd got it all ready for you first,' she fired back.

Tonight Annie is tucking into a vast tub of pasta and working on the phones when I arrive. I don't get the chance to do much more than smile a quick hello. I clock on just before six, do a bit of admin then head off for my first, surprisingly early house-call at half past.

My first driver of the night is Roger. I take a deep breath and try not to catch Annie's eye as I follow him to the car park. Roger is one of the nicest guys you could meet – and one of the worst drivers. He's never had a crash. He doesn't double the speed limit. But he does turn a simple journey into something akin to a theme park ride. Some of the doctors will feign anything to avoid going on a call with him. 'I don't care how ill the patients are. If Roger's driving I'll be too sick to treat them,' one of my fellow GPs likes to say. Tonight I'm hoping that early rush hour traffic means he won't be able to do more than crawl through the streets. I'm wrong. The roads seem to open up ahead of us. We lurch wildly round what should be perfectly ordinary corners as we head east. Roger appears to misunderstand the whole concept of mini-roundabouts and speed bumps as he bounces us towards the car roof and does some serious damage to the suspension. Amber lights at pedestrian crossings appear to be a particular issue for him. On-coming traffic seems to be a personal affront.

A journey that should normally take twenty minutes takes less than ten. That's the one saving grace of Roger's driving.

Journeys always end sooner than you predict. 'This is it, boss,' he says cheerfully as he slices between some parked cars outside a tall residential tower. I grab my bag, steady myself the way you do when you get off a boat, and head towards the buzzers at the communal doors.

'I'm … getting … scared … now,' the woman says from the bed in front of me. She's taking shallow, bubbling breaths that clearly alarm the heck out of her. The room's incredibly warm. She's propped up on a whole load of cushions and pillows and she's got wide, terrified eyes. They close, squeezing out tears, as her left hand snakes surprisingly quickly across to my arm. She grips it, tighter than you'd ever imagine. She's Indian, in her late seventies and she's got end-stage heart failure. We've got plenty of information on her. Her surgery had flagged her up as someone who might need home visits at night. Her notes are detailed and comprehensive. Her care has been good. But her prospects are poor.

I ask a few questions and check a few details – but in reality there's very little extra I need to know and very little extra I can do. This is yet another family who want their mum to stay at home. It is another occasion when I agree with them.

'I can give her something to help settle her anxiety. That should help with her breathing and take the edge off any pain,' I say quietly. I administer the drug and talk the son through a few other issues. Patients in this condition can benefit from some diuretics as well. Fluid can build up in the lungs at this stage of the game. It triggers this lady's characteristic bubbling breath. It can make you panic as you feel as if you're drowning – and it can sound like a real death rattle that can scare the heck out of patient and family alike. Diuretics can help reduce the problem with the fluid build-up – but they can also trigger kidney problems. As usual at this stage of an illness we're between a rock and a hard place. The treatment for one condition can bring forward another. That dilemma is even more pronounced with medications like diamorphine. It can calm patients down and take away the panic that's overwhelmed them. But it can, of course, take them closer to the end as well. That's life – and death – in a nutshell for medics. Sometimes you have to accept that while a drug is given for a positive reason it will have a negative effect as well. That's the tightrope everyone has to walk.

'She'll sleep soon and she'll be calm for a while,' I say quietly as the lady's family gather around.

'Thank you so much,' says her son. 'She was really suffering earlier on.'

I collect my things and get ready to leave when he stops me.

'I think my mother wants to speak to you before you go,' he says. I turn back to the bed. The lady has stopped crying and looks calm at last. Her face is weak but she is using her eyes to motion me towards her. She opens her mouth to try to speak but the words don't come. Then her hand reaches out towards me one last time. She pats my arm very lightly three times. She gives a half smile. Then she turns her head slightly into her pillows and closes her eyes.

'I think she just wanted to say thanks,' the man says quietly. I tell him she didn't need to and take my leave. This is one of the hard parts of life as a sessional doctor, especially at night. If you make a real effort you can follow cases up and find out how patients are doing and whether their conditions improve. I do sometimes check that referrals or tests or daytime appointments are made. But a lot of the time you're a one hit wonder.

You come into people's lives at their most vulnerable moments. You meet families amidst scenes of absolute distress. And you don't know how their stories end. In cases like this though, you can have a pretty good guess.

Chapter Three:

Time for a Moan

I'm doing a six-hour, early-evening shift for one of the big, outsourced companies tonight – so most of the faces are new to me. We're typically United Nations, like so much of the NHS in London. Both our nurses and one of our doctors are Spanish and our other doctor is Estonian. On a smaller scale, even our drivers are diverse. We've got two Scots, a Geordie and a man in a Manchester United shirt. As a lifelong Blackburn Rovers fan I take an instant dislike to him. But I hope we do a job together. I'll enjoy taking him back a few years and reminding him of 1995.

But back to the doctors – and to one of the big worries we've all got about the job. Over the years we've all worked with people whose English doesn't stretch particularly far. If they came to Britain on holiday they'd be fine ordering a meal or getting directions to the London Eye. But speaking to and understanding sick and scared patients in the small hours of the morning? Verbal and social skills are vital if GPs are to do their jobs right. We can't diagnose safely without them. We learn from the things patients don't say, just as much as from what they do. We pick up on nuances and silences. We need to understand our patients on an awful lot of levels. In short, we need to truly speak their language.

So why does Britain employ doctors who struggle to understand their patients? I don't know. But employ them we do. Every time there's a scandal – or, worse, a death – involving an overseas doctor the Government of the day acts shocked and promises immediate reform. Then everything goes quiet.

One last thought before I stop my rant. I did French and German at school about twenty years ago. About five years ago I decided to learn Italian. I spent about a week listening to a CD then gave up. On the back of those very limited language skills let's say I call up some agency in Paris, Berlin or Rome and applied to work night shifts in one of their busiest areas. I'd fall off my chair if they offered me a job and let me loose on their sick citizens. I cannot believe that the governments of France, Germany or Italy would let a non-native speaker fly in to do such a vital job. If EU law says they've got to employ me then I cannot believe the French, for example, would cave in and comply with it. I bet they protect their citizens by putting up some hurdle – a hurdle, like, oh I don't know, a proper language test.

Meanwhile we've done the opposite in Britain. We fill gaps by welcoming foreign doctors with open arms and open chequebooks. They're decent people, for the most part. Marko, who I've met for the first time tonight, is personable, keen and efficient. He's just the sort of doctor I'd like looking after me if I fell ill in his native Estonia.

Thousands of miles from Estonia I do worry about it all, sometimes. We all know doctors who've skipped or even failed language tests and aren't up to speed on all the different drugs we prescribe in the UK.

Hopefully this madness is starting to end. There's a big movement towards local GPs for local patients – and in big cities like London it's starting to get results. The Spanish GP I'm working with has lived here for years and I'd trust her with anyone and anything. The more recent and less settled arrivals are a bit more of a worry. On a national level we're told that language tests for EU doctors are under consideration once again. There's also talk of proper induction programmes for overseas doctors. We're told that consultations are going on, reports will be published and appropriate action will be taken. But in the meantime I sit here, in London, with Marko at my side. He's young and newly qualified so with a bit of luck his medical skills will be top notch. But we sit in silence because we've pretty much exhausted our limited common conversation. Maybe I'll be wrong about the implications of all this. Maybe an Estonian patient who doesn't speak a word of English will call out a GP and Marko will save the day. Maybe.

Chapter Four:

The Early Hours

Vincent looks perfectly well as he walks into my surgery. Perfectly well but very sheepish. He takes off his shirt, lifts up his arms and I soon see why.

'Oh dear. What have you been up to?' I ask, with a bit of a grimace.

'I was using my girlfriend's wax stuff,' he begins. 'I wanted to see what it would look like.'

'And your test area was the whole of both underarms?' I ask with a bit of a smile.

'I should probably have read the instructions a bit better,' he admits.

He certainly should. When he pulled off the wax he somehow managed to pull off whole chunks of skin as well. Most people would have stopped at that point. Vincent must have carried on pulling. Several colours of the rainbow show through the weeping wounds he's created. The pain must be searing through him. The healing process will take quite some time – and the risk is that a secondary infection like cellulitis creeps in before it's done. I glove up, get a sterile tray ready and lean in to clean up the wounds. It's not the most exciting medical job in the world. Most nights this would probably be done by one of the nurses but all of them must be busy so I'm happy to get the job done myself.

'I'm guessing it said to leave the wax on for two minutes or something? And you left it on for what, twenty?' I ask as I bathe the edge of the wound and watch a grown man try very hard not to cry.

'I wanted to make sure it was done,' he says, staring fixedly at the surgery wall ahead of him. 'The only good news is that I started out on my underarms. I was going to do my balls.'

We talk about everything and nothing as I clean and dress the wounds. I give him a prescription to stop infection, tell him to read the instructions properly this time and take the full course. Then I head to reception to get a coffee and watch him join his very beautiful girlfriend in the waiting area. She looks a little bit concerned and a whole lot amused. I doubt this poor guy will be allowed to forget tonight in a hurry.

It's just gone two in the morning. My shift tonight had begun at midnight and the OOH centre I'm part of is right alongside one of the big hospitals. It's in a set of rooms in a portacabin in the car park, to be exact. That means it would be easy to point a lot of patients across the car park and into A&E. We could do that whenever we get someone particularly tricky in our surgery. That way they magically become someone else's problem for the night. I've winced after seeing some of my fellow locums do just that. I try not to. We're in a sort of grey area of the health service. Very few of the A&E staff will ever get to meet us. Some of them might not know that we set up camp in spare rooms in their hospital grounds every night. But they'd soon get wise if we stopped pulling our weight. There are some feisty A&E managers in London who would come marching round pretty fast to read us the riot act and tell us to do our jobs rather than adding to theirs. I'd be mortified if that happened when I was on a shift. I want a good reputation not a bad name. Consultants and hospital doctors spend enough time bad mouthing GPs as it is. They are always saying we're only good at the fluffy, hand-holding side of medicine. I want to prove them wrong.

Tonight my other big goal is to get something to eat. The good thing about working a night shift on hospital premises is that you can sometimes sneak off for some food. It might just be a vending machine, but it's better than nothing.

I get back to base with a very healthy meal of crisps and chocolate and everyone wants to share it. We've hit a quiet patch. Our other GP is out on calls, a few calls need to be returned but none have been flagged as urgent. So the nurses, the drivers and I kick back for a bit. We have a bit of a laugh about a recent report into the service we provide out of hours. A survey has thrown up a litany of supposedly shocking accusations. One family had issued an official complaint because they suspected that the doctor who had answered their house-call had been – wait for it – chewing gum. Then there was the patient who demanded a house-call because they were in too much pain to sleep. Apparently they then nodded off and complained when the GP arrived and woke them up by ringing the door bell. Several others complained that the doctor sent out in the early hours to help them had – in their opinion – lacked empathy, been distant or impatient. I wish them well with an overly chummy alternative who invades their personal space and hangs around in their kitchen all night drinking tea.

Still, it could be worse. We could be across the way in A&E. We've not got the latest on what their patients are complaining about. But we've got plenty of anecdotes about the ridiculous things that are happening in their world. Annie repeats the story about the perfectly fit and healthy guy in the Midlands who bought a milkshake at McDonalds, thought it smelt a bit off, so took it to A&E and expected the staff to analyse it for him. Someone else remembers the man who went to hospital when the batteries in his hearing aid needed to be changed.

When the crisps and chocolate are all gone I head back to the phones for a while. I advise a few people to come in to see us, but most of the other callers are sorted out with a bit of advice and reassurance. And between each call I stand up and walk around a bit. The walls in our portacabin don't just let in the cold – they seem to magnify it. They do the same to the noise as the car park outside slowly fills up for the day ahead.

I think about a friend of mine in Manchester whose OOH shifts are based in a quite extraordinarily well-resourced sexual health centre he claims has original art on the walls, fresh flowers on the tables and ceiling-high, multi-coloured glass sculptures beside the reception desk. Lots of surveys show that the better a patient's surroundings the better his or her health outcome will be. But floor-to-ceiling glass sculptures?

Waste, duplication and misdirected resources are just three of the dirty little secrets in the NHS. But in an organisation that's supposed to be one of the biggest single employers in the world, right up there with the Chinese army or the Indian railways, I imagine things won't always be as tight or well managed as they could be. And unless selling off the art in the Midlands gets me an air heater or a better coffee machine in south east London then patients might as well enjoy the sculptures while they can.

I follow Annie's lead and put my coat on at my computer as I do a bit of admin. I imagine that the actual handover process varies in different centres and in different parts of the country – but that's the vast, unwieldy NHS for you again. With luck, once I've put something on to the computer it's automatically faxed to patients' surgeries to be scanned in or otherwise updated on their next business day. Surgery staff get the consultation details including the presenting complaint, the history of it, examination details, diagnosis, treatment and details of any necessary follow-ups and clinical codes. They update their patients' records accordingly so everyone knows who has been seen and why. It's important for patients' long-term care, obviously. It's just as important if we're to stop patients from playing the system and getting medication they don't need or shouldn't have.

Record keeping is very repetitive, because the rules demand it and because doctors spend an awful lot of time worrying about being sued. That's why we have more than a paper trail to follow. Calls are recorded, right from the start, and transcripts can be dredged up for years afterwards if required. Regardless of the process, the theory is that full details of any work we do at night will soon go on your file. When I've got the last of my night's admin done I have a final chat with Annie and some of the drivers and watch as the surgery clock ticks towards eight. At that point the computer system will automatically switch off our phones. Call your local surgery now and you'll go right through to your usual reception staff. It's time for us to go to bed.

Chapter Five:

I'm Not Your Friend

It's one o'clock in the morning. My colleague Anil is out in the car doing home visits. I'm seeing patients back at base. The next of them is a 22-year-old man. He bounces into my surgery – almost literally. He's skinny as a rake and high as a kite. Oh, and he's got company. Another lad, probably a bit younger, is with him.

'My mate needs Valium, dude,' the younger man says.

I bite my lip. I'm not a stand-on-ceremony sort of person. I don't expect people to defer to me or call me 'Doctor' all the time. But 'Dude'? This isn't southern California. We're not surfers. And we're certainly not friends.

'I'm Doctor Rudd,' I say firmly and turn to the sky-high guy. 'What's your name and what's the problem?' I've got his details on my screen but I want to see how aware and responsive he is.

He tells me, his face cracking open in a huge smile, his eyes darting all over the surgery, every part of his body flinching and fidgeting, jolting and jerking all at once. He's utterly agitated.

He is happy as anything, but right on the edge and well out of control.

'We've been at a club. Two clubs. We've done some stuff. He won't come down, dunno why. He needs Valium. I've seen it done before. It'll bring him down,' the friend interrupts.

'What do you mean by stuff?'

'Coke.'

I tap some details into the computer. I hate the fact that the guy is very probably right about what's needed. For some reason I've dealt with a lot more heroin addicts than cocaine cases over the years. Like most night-time GPs I've seen my fair share of methadone as well – and I know from friends in A&E that a lot of the newer legal highs are causing a whole slew of new problems. But I don't think I've ever seen anyone trip quite like this from coke. I do know, though, what has to be done. I ask a few more questions and check a few more physical features. The man is heating up a little too nicely, his heartbeat is racing and his blood pressure is high. Worst-case scenario is that he could have anything from a stroke to a cerebral haemorrhage. So I bow to the inevitable. I prescribe a one-off dose of valium – and I make the patient swallow it in front of me. Both guys seem to think the whole thing is funny. I just think it's sad.

I've always been a bit zero tolerant of drugs. I see the damage they can do to people's health and I sense the wider damage they do to society. Years ago, to keep an ex-girlfriend happy, I kept silent when a group of her supposedly well-educated, middle class friends called some dealer to get a bit of Friday night cocaine – then proceeded to moan that they'd had their car broken into and that their neighbourhood was over-run by a criminal underclass.

As doctors we can't be judgemental about our patients – and I'm not a naturally judgemental person to start with. But part of our job is to guide people towards a healthier life. Full time GPs tie themselves up in knots trying to meet government targets by identifying smokers, drinkers and the obese without 'stigmatising' patients for, well, smoking, drinking and refusing to get off the sofa.

I'm free of most of that bureaucracy as a sessional, out-of-hours doctor. But I do have opinions. I'd certainly hazard a guess that this guy's life would be a whole lot healthier if he gave up the drugs and ate a few proper meals. If I had to give him social advice I'd also suggest he find better friends. So do I say it? I decide not to waste my breath – and it seems the appointment isn't quite over.

'Any chance of a taxi home? We're in the middle of nowhere here,' the kid says as his mate gets up to leave.

I don't even acknowledge him. 'Just close the door on your way out,' I say. Dude.

Chapter Six:

Other Addicts

Do we really need GPs to be on call all night at all? If your life is in danger you 999 your way to hospital – and if it it's not then you can wait till the morning, right?

Well, maybe. There's a huge grey area between those two extremes. Lots of conditions are urgent but not emergencies. A big part of what we do at night is to stop the former from turning into the latter. And if we can keep people at home and keep them healthy till morning we can save the NHS a whole lot of cash. We stop A&E from breaching its waiting targets and filling up expensive hospital beds. And, of course, we help people.

The number of house-calls we do varies hugely. In some parts of the country two in ten calls to an OOH centre trigger a home visit. In others it's two in a hundred. I suppose it all depends on how the initial calls are answered and who does the triage. A lot of the house-calls are pretty routine. All some people need is a doctor to check up on them. In a perfect world it would be their usual GP, the friendly face they see all the time who knows everything about them and their condition. In reality it's going to be someone like me, or someone like me from overseas, who needs a bit of extra cash but doesn't know the patient from Adam.

The good news is that a fresh pair of eyes can sometimes be exactly what's required. I've done my share of full-time, daytime surgeries over the years. I know how easy it is to be blinded by our most regular patients. They are the ones who turn up week in and week out to raise the same old issues. The ones where we've heard all the symptoms a hundred times before and where we decide how each consultation should end before it's fully begun. Throw a brand new GP into the mix, in the middle of the night, and the picture can be quite different. The new GP hasn't got any baggage. So once in a blue moon he or she might see or hear something that's been overlooked.

The bad news is that the lack of baggage can turn out to be a distinct disadvantage. Most people think that we'll have your full, vital medical history at our fingertips when we reach your bedside. Sometimes we don't even know how to spell your name. I read someone's description of out-of-hours GPs the other day. 'We regularly assess unknown and acutely unwell patients without access to their medical records,' it began. It doesn't inspire much confidence, I know. Obviously A&E staff don't have access to people's medical records either, when seriously ill trauma patients get stretchered in after a blue-light dash across town. But at least A&E staff have each other. We tend to be on our own, in people's houses, at 3am. So the occasional clue about your patient's past medical history wouldn't go amiss. But how can we get it?

The computerisation of the NHS is a very sore and very expensive subject. Of course it makes sense to encourage it. It's staggering that some close-to-retirement, one-man-band GP practices in the capital and elsewhere are still run with barely a nod to new technology. Of course there are huge issues about confidentiality and access that have to be addressed. And getting different systems to talk to each other is incredibly expensive – or so the teams of shiny young management consultants always tell us.

Tonight's one of the nights when a bit of background is certainly required. I'm driven off to an address way out west in Gunnersbury. It's just gone ten and the patient says he's run out of his anti-depressant medication. He's 33, angry, agitated and says he doesn't know what he might do if I don't help him. His plan is for me to write him out an emergency prescription to give him a whole lot of new pills. In your dreams, mate, I say to myself as he tries to make his case. For I'm pretty certain this patient has been down this road before.

Benzo addicts – people on drugs like diazepam and temazepam – are as sneaky as any other addict. The more desperate they become the sneakier they try to be. I've had middle-aged women claiming they need prescriptions for fake sisters with non-existent cancers. I've had people self-harm and say they've been mugged for their meds and need a new supply fast. Sometimes the stories can be pretty good. But desperation normally shows in peoples' eyes.

I carry on with a few basic questions.

'Because I've lost my effing prescription,' he yells at me when I ask him yet again why I'm there.

'I thought you said you'd run out of your prescription?'

'What's the difference? Just write me out a new one. I'm on the edge here. It'll be on your record if I do something bad tonight.'

'When did you last take the medication?'

'I don't remember. That's why I effing need it.'

'Yesterday? The day before? More than a week ago? Or did you take it as normal today?'

He's wound up like a clock now. It's pretty clear I'm not the doctor he was hoping to meet. After a whole lot more pointless argy-bargy I make him my final offer. I'll prescribe him a single dose, enough to get him through to the morning when he can try it on with his regular GP.

'I can't get to see my regular GP! Have you ever tried to get an appointment? That's why I've called you. That's what this is all about.'

I'm glad he said that. Because I enjoy replying to that one. 'You don't get a house-call from an out-of-hours GP just because you can't be bothered to go to your local surgery like everyone else. That is not how this works. I can inform your local surgery and they'll know to expect you first thing. But this is all you're getting from me.' I write out my single dose prescription. He refuses to take it.

'And I've got to go and get the pills myself? In the middle of the night?' he asks, outraged. I don't bother to reply. If I was being really tough I could make him get the medication and take it in front of me. Directly observed dosing is one of the things that's used to make sure people on medication like methadone aren't just collecting the pills then selling them on. Not that DOD is entirely fool proof. We all know stories about desperate druggies swallowing their dose on cue – then disappearing to a toilet or a doorway to try and vomit it up into a plastic bag. The pill in that bag, vomit and all, gets sold to someone who's even more desperate and the whole cycle of addictive misery continues.

Tonight I don't judge that this guy needs policing and I don't think I'm creating a secondary market in bags full of vomit. My assessment is that the drugs are for himself, not for sale. All I need do now is get my message across and get on with my job.

'Do you want the prescription or not?' I ask.

'I want a full course,' he says very slowly and deliberately. Threats are flashing in his eyes. This is getting interesting. 'Doctors have given that to me at night before.'

'I don't care,' I tell him. 'Like I say, you can't use us to get medication at night that you wouldn't get in the day. You won't get away with it.'

'I will. And one day some little girl or some foreigner will give me what I want.' He looks as if he's building up to spit at me. I stand forward and will him to go ahead and do it. That way I can call the police, get all this properly recorded and make his future a whole lot more complicated.

The man turns away. Perhaps he's not quite as stupid as he looks. 'No one, no doctor, will ever prescribe you what you want,' I tell the man as I leave. I speak with absolute, unshakeable certainty. If only I believed it.

Chapter Seven:

The Man at the Table

There's another reason why out of hours GP services are so important at night – because nights are when an awful lot of people die. This isn't how we come into the world. I'm not certain, but I'm pretty sure that births are spread pretty equally through all 24 hours. There are several theories about why death is different – not least that it's all down to the circadian rhythms that are supposed to govern everything from people to plants.

Whatever the reason, countless older people wake up to find their partners have died, next to them, in the marital bed they've shared for so many years. At medical school I used to think that must be the saddest thing in the world. I used to think you couldn't recover from that shock. I thought that you'd have to move house to cast out the terrible memories.

Then I went out there and began to examine and certify the death of people who had passed away in that fashion. I began to meet the wives and sometimes the husbands who had woken up alone. I realised that when you truly love someone you can put their feelings ahead of your grief. You can be glad for them, not sorry for yourself. You can be glad that they passed away in peace and without pain. You can be glad that they died in the place and next to the person that they too loved. That's your comfort. It's the thing you can cling to and focus upon. At some point in the future I want a wife and kids. Even further ahead, as long as our kids are grown-up and safe, I'd like my wife and I to die at the exact same time. As that probably won't happen I don't know which of us I'd like to go first. But I do know that the peace of the night would be a good time for the first of us to say a silent goodbye.

It's just after nine on a busy Saturday night when we get a call to verify a slightly different death on our patch.

It's a Mr James Sylvester, a retired caretaker with a dodgy ticker and a long history of ill health. He was alive and as well as could be expected when his wife headed off to see her daughter on Friday morning – and he was very clearly dead on her return the following evening. The couple's house, a smart terrace in the middle of a shabby warren of streets in Southwark, is very full and very noisy when we arrive.

'It was my granddad. My gran, my mum and I found him. I was going to do that thing to his chest but he was dead and my mum said not to touch him. I did though. He was really, really cold. He'd been dead for ages. He'd not eaten any of the food my gran had left for him on Friday. She's not taking it very well,' a lad of about fifteen says in a mad rush at the door. The words have tumbled out of him and his face and his eyes are full of emotion. There's a worry there, a concern and a sadness. But there's also a flash of pride at his own role in the night's events. He's clearly taken some sort of control of the situation.

By 'that thing to his chest' I assume he means CPR. I was first taught that as a kid at Scouts. Do London kids go to Scouts any more? Or did he learn it in school? Either way, all credit to him for being ready to use it on his granddad. Doing CPR on a real body, cracking the ribs of someone you know and love, is very different to doing it on a funny-looking plastic torso in a classroom. The adrenaline flows for some time afterwards, even for us.

'It sounds like you've done the right thing,' I tell him to his obvious pleasure. 'Can you take me to your grandfather's body?'

He nods. But before we take more than a couple of steps, there's a huge wail of anguish from the room to our left.

'That's my gran,' the lad says, looking uncertain.

The wail echoes down the hall again. It descends into a whole orchestra of sobbing.

'I'll see your gran first,' I say. In cases like this we owe a duty of care to the living, as well as a responsibility to the dead. It's never easy walking into a house full of grieving, angry, confused or guilt-ridden relatives. But it's a big part of the job.

'Mrs Sylvester? I'm Doctor Rudd. I'm very sorry for your loss.' I'm not sure you can beat the standard phrases at times like this. The very fact that they are almost clichés can bring a level of normality to the situation.

Tonight, though, Mrs Sylvester isn't ready to hear them.

She's a small, tightly wound woman in her mid-sixties. She's pacing a patch of thickly carpeted floor in front of the home's bay window. She's shaking and her hands are raking through her short, white hair. Two women, who I assume must be her daughters, are trying to hold her still and sit her back down.

'The doctor's here, mum. You have to listen to him,' says one. There are tears in her own eyes.

'Mrs Sylvester, why don't you sit down for me? Just for a moment so I can check you're OK,' I say.

And sit she does. She slumps, very suddenly, into what looks like the least comfortable armchair in the world. She puts her face in her hands. She breathes hard and a lot of time seems to pass. Then she looks right at me.

'I loved him,' she says. Three little words. 'I loved him and I don't know what I'll do without him.' She adds. Her eyes lose their focus as the first edges of grief approach. She stays silent as her daughters reach over and hold her hands. The room is calm at last. She'll be OK for now.

'I'll be back in a moment,' I say. It's time to see the body. Connor is hovering by the door and leads me through the house to the kitchen.

A man is standing awkwardly by a spotlessly clean sink. 'I'm Gemma's husband. I'm his son-in-law,' he says. I introduce myself, put down my medical bag and start work.

I take a quick look around. Mr Sylvester's death counts as expected because of his long standing ill health. But you want to be sure he wasn't helped on his way. You want to check everything looks the way it should. Tonight it does. His body is at the kitchen table. A thick skin floats on top of a half-drunk mug of milky coffee to his side. The sports pages of yesterday's Daily Mail are open in front of him. His head is bowed and the muscles in his face have relaxed. He is, indeed, very cold.

I start my examination. It sounds a bit odd, but it begins by checking the patient really is dead. Mistakes have happened in the past – stories about this kind of thing are told all the time. When I've established death tonight I look all around the man's body, his face and his neck. 'Nobody's moved him. We thought that was best,' the man says as I attempt to lift one of Mr Sylvester's arms.

'That's good, thank you,' I reply automatically. The man's arm is stiff. If death occurred yesterday morning then that's to be expected. A few more hours – normally from about 36 hours after death – and bodies change again and go flaccid.

One of the daughters comes into the room and I ask her a few details about her dad's recent health and record all the facts I need. I'm not issuing what's commonly known as a death certificate. The rules on those are deliberately tough – mainly due to common sense, best practice and Harold Shipman. In simple terms, doctors can only sign them if they've seen the patient alive in the past two weeks. That's not normally going to include occasional night-time GPs like me. My task is really just to verify that the man is dead, at which point the undertakers can remove the body. As the death was expected, and as long as there are no suspicions, his regular GP can certify the death tomorrow and the family can take the next steps and have it registered.

I put my paperwork back in my bag and head back to check up on Mrs Sylvester. She's still quiet. She's moved from the arm chair and is sitting at a dining table at the back of the room. I'm sure she won't realise it, but she's in exactly the same position as her late husband.

'Is there anything you want to ask, or anything I can tell you before I go?' I ask, taking a chair opposite her.

There isn't. But there's something she wants to say to me. 'I wasn't with him,' she says after a while. 'I spent the night with our daughter's family. I was only in Sevenoaks. I wasn't far. But I wasn't here.'

'You got back this evening?' I ask. It's useful background, but it's also clear that it will help this lady to talk. Answering a few questions will see her through a few more moments. It will give her a bit of space to regroup.

'Maggie drove me. Connor came along for the ride. He went into the kitchen first. He found him. He dialled 999 and they told him what to do.'

Her voice breaks so I interrupt. 'Connor did really well. You should be very proud of him.'

Mrs Sylvester smiles, a sudden, unexpected smile that fades as fast as it came. Her mind, clearly, has gone straight back to her late husband. 'He was exactly where I left him yesterday morning,' she says, a dreamy quality in her voice. 'I made him that cup of coffee before I left. I put my hand on his shoulder as I left the room. Since he retired he's sat in that chair every morning to read the paper and do the crossword. He must have died the moment I left the house.'

'There's no sign of any trauma. He may well have nodded off and died in his sleep,' I tell her.

'Everyone loved him, doctor,' she says, suddenly defensive. 'He had so many friends. He'd have gone for a walk later. He'd have smiled at people, said hello. Everyone loved him, doctor. We loved him.' There's an edge of hysteria in her voice again but she quells it. She sits there, twisting her wedding ring round her finger, looking blankly into the distance. 'Forty eight years. We were married for forty eight years,' she says eventually. The tears are back now. Her daughters move just a little closer.

'Your husband didn't suffer,' I repeat. But other than that I just sit very still for a few moments. Doctors occupy a very odd place in these situations. Humanity can tell us that the one thing some people need is to be held or to be hugged. Some doctors might do that. I'm sorry, but I tend to hold back. Sometimes I judge that I can't reach out a comforting arm, let alone allow someone to cry on my shoulder. I might be wrong, but I feel it blurs the line between doctor and patient, it raises too many issues and it risks breaking too many rules. Anyway, tonight Mrs Sylvester has plenty of family and friends around to hold her. She doesn't need me for that. She needs me to be a doctor.

'Mrs Sylvester your husband won't have suffered. He was at home, reading the paper. He would have been happy,' I repeat. Then I explain a little more about undertakers and paperwork, what will happen next. Mrs Sylvester nods and appears to brace herself for the challenge. I stand up, watch as her daughters move in for that long overdue hug, then I take my leave. Connor is standing in the hall, eyes bright looking like the man of the house. Another elderly lady, a neighbour or a friend, has just arrived and he is guiding her towards his gran. As I leave the house, and look around, I see that it is still one of the few homes on the street with lights in its windows. It's full of life, even in death.

Chapter Eight:

Breathing Easy as Night

I'M back doing a night shift at one of the best GP co-operatives way out east. A fair few of my favourite faces are there and as we're relatively quiet we have plenty of time to chat between appointments. We've also got time to bend the rules if required. That's why Annie comes into my room just after half past four in the morning. The wire from her phone headset is trailing behind her, making her look like something from a sci-fi film. If I was quick-witted enough I'd have a funny line to say about it. Instead I ask what she wants.

'I've taken pity on someone. He's a really nice man. Can you give him a quick call?' she says, handing me a print-out of a name and number.

'Hello there, I'm Doctor Rudd from the out-of-hours service. How can I help?'

'Thank you so much for calling back. I can't quite believe I've had to ask this. But I'm at the end of my tether.' The man proceeds, very clearly, to explain. He's a police officer. Every few years he's had major foot pain that he is convinced is gout, though it's never been properly diagnosed. He's 44, fit and healthy and doesn't fit into any key risk-categories but it strikes him all the same. Three hours ago he says he was woken up by his latest attack.

'It was everything I've had before and more. Just incredible, bizarre pain in my right big toe. So painful that you can't even have the sheet on it, just the way they always describe it. Incredible that such a tiny part of your body can hurt so much. I'd forgotten how bad it is.'

'It certainly sounds like something you should see your GP about in the morning,' I begin. I'm sympathetic but careful. You don't need urgent care just because your toe hurts.

'I would do, of course,' the man says. 'I'm ringing now because I've got a training day that starts at eight. It's mandatory attendance. I can't miss it and I won't be able to take part – and I might not be able to get there – if my foot stays this bad. I've got three kids at home. Their mum's not here and we're on our own till seven so there's no-one to look after them if I get a taxi to A&E. I need something to calm my foot down for the morning so I can do my course. I'll see my GP as soon as I can. But I'm desperate right now. It's embarrassing and I feel an idiot. But I need help.'

I tell him we'll happily see him in the centre and I hear him sigh.

'I just don't know what to do about the kids. I can't think who I can get round to look after them at this time in the morning,' he begins.

'How old are they?'

'Evan's eighteen months, Ben's three and Izzy is five.'

'Well bring them with you. They'll be looked after while we see you. There's a play area and everything here,' I say.

'Tell him we've got chocolate biscuits,' Annie mouths. She's been standing close and listening in on the call. I know she's got a bit of a soft spot for police and other emergency service workers – honour among thieves and all that.

I ignore her. 'Is there anyone you can call to sit with them? A neighbour? The kids' grandparents? Is your wife due back in the morning?'

There's another long pause. 'My wife's actually with you guys. She's in hospital. She's at the Marsden. It's cervical cancer. We're having a bit of a bad year.'

I put the man on hold for a moment and check the situation with Annie. Our call-backs are pretty much up to date, she says, our other GPs are both in the base and our drivers are twiddling their thumbs in the coffee room. We'd never normally do a home visit for something as trivial as this but we're able to show discretion when family circumstances are particularly tough. I think we should do so tonight. I log off my computer and set off on a quick visit. Not that there's much I can do. The guy has been online and read about joint injections and steroid treatments but I have to tell him they won't help. After a quick examination and a few questions all I can do is offer him the strongest anti-inflammatories around and tell him to see his regular GP about long term preventative treatment. We talk very briefly about his wife and how their kids are coping then I head back to the car. However useless it was, I'm glad I did the visit. And it seems I've another one lined up.

Roger passes over the details as I swing myself into the passenger seat. Fortunately we've not got far to go. The OOH service does try to batch local calls together to make best use of everyone's time at night and stop the same doctors criss-crossing each other in the early hours. Some nights it works well – and I can spend three or four hours of a shift in the car doing back-to-back calls. Other nights it falls apart a bit and we seem to waste a lot of time and petrol going back to base all the time.

Tonight this latest call is for a woman in her early seventies. She's got chronic obstructive pulmonary disease or COPD. It's a very common form of permanent lung damage that can be treated but can't be cured. You end up suffering from breathlessness, inflammation, endless coughing and you have an awful lot of mucus to shift around your airways. This lady has asthma as well – so it's probably been a very long time since she breathed easy.

She lives on her own so after her latest attack she's struggled to the front door, taken a gamble by leaving it ajar, then slumped in an armchair in her lounge. Elderly people with COPD – especially the lifelong smokers – can be incredibly brittle. This lady bears very little resemblance to Venus de Milo. But she does look as if bits of her might break off at any moment.

'Thank you for coming. You're an angel. Thank you, sweetheart,' she says between coughs and gasps. She gives it everything to try and give me a big smile as well.

I get to work. I like this lady's spirit but I am worried about her health.

I start off by taking her pulse. Anything over 100 will be a bad sign, but she's not quite there yet. I ask her when the latest attack began. If she can't complete a sentence then that's bad too. She just about makes it, though her gasps for breath are worthy of a 70's horror film. I clip a pulse oximeter on to her finger to measure her oxygen saturation. It's low, but not too low. Mrs Warne is in a bad way, but it could be a lot worse. It's time to fix her.

'Let's get you sorted. You've done all this before, have you?' I ask.

The lady nods, between another orchestral burst of coughs and gasps. I get her a glass of water from her kitchen and hand her some steroid tablets. They should start to calm some of the inflammation in her airways and allow a little more air to her lungs. Then it's time for the nebuliser. I've brought it in from the car and get it ready for action. Nebulisers help get medication direct to a patient's lungs by issuing it in a fine mist. They've got their downsides and they're noisy as anything but they're just what Mrs Warne requires right now. I hand her a face mask, check everything is connected and wait to see if her condition improves or whether she's going to need more care in hospital.

'Feeling a little easier?' I ask after five or so minutes. She nods an emphatic 'yes' through the mask. She holds it off her face for a moment and flashes me a hopeful smile. Then she grips it back to suck in every moment of aid. A further five or so minutes down the line it's clear she's going in the right direction.

She's ready and able to talk so I start to ask her a few questions about her health and her care. She interrupts me.

'Doctor, I'm so sorry, but I've been sat here so long and I'm gasping for the loo,' she says.

I support her as she struggles the short distance down the hall to her bathroom. I wait outside to take her back to her chair. 'That's made everything better. I thought I might forget myself if I stayed in that chair a moment longer,' she admits with a cough and a bit of a fruity laugh, as she settles back down.

That crisis averted she runs through all the people who usually help her. The community air team are on her case and while she can't quite master their jargon it seems as if a ceiling of care has been agreed and lots of worst-case scenarios have been discussed. It's equally clear that a lot of work has been done to ensure she can stay at home for as long as possible. She's got a portable oxygen cylinder next to her chair and on the table in front of her is a shop-load of inhalers and other kit. She's lucid and almost lively again now. But will she be OK till morning?

People with COPD can be a tough call at night. They can go off fast. You need to be sure they don't have chest infections or even pneumonia. I listen to her chest but I can't hear any problems. My judgement is that Mrs Warne can stay right where she is. If her breathing gets bad again she could go to hospital and go on a ventilator. But that can be a one way street with the elderly. Once they're on a ventilator that's often where they stay. They might even get polished off by a hospital infection. Survive that and the stress of hospitalisation, plus the worry about your home and all the things you've left behind, can trigger an asthma attack. An A&E trip would cost the NHS a fortune, take up a valuable bed, ruin Mrs Warne's night and put a big question mark over her future. All things considered I think this jolly old lady is better off where she is.

I'm particularly confident in my diagnosis because Mrs Warne's recovery is gaining pace. She's calmer and a whole lot more comfortable. She's also incredibly grateful for my help. I ask if there's anyone who can sit with her till morning and she swears she'll be fine on her own. She offers me a coffee and says she's got a new packet of shortbread in the kitchen. I judge that she's OK. But I can't leave without telling her off.

'You're still smoking, aren't you love?' I ask, looking at the stubs in the ash tray beside her chair.

'I try, doctor, I try. But I just can't stop,' she says sheepishly.

'Do you need me to give you another lecture? To tell you that smoking is making these attacks more frequent? Do you want me to tell you where you can get help giving up?'

She's got a real twinkle in her eye now. She understands me, which is nice. And she clearly is feeling much better, which is even nicer. 'I think the last doctor did all that,' she says.

'And the one before?'

'And the one before that.'

'Well one day you should listen to us. Otherwise you'll hurt our feelings.'

I head outside and Roger drives me back to base, treating the streets of suburban south London like the final lap at Le Mans. Everything is still pretty quiet at the health centre. Some nights are like this. One of the GPs has a patient in his room and Annie is on the phone. She's rolling her eyes as she tries to focus on what seems to be a long-running conversation with someone who thinks their bad back is caused by sneezing – and wants to know what we're going to do about it. The rest of the team is in the kitchen area drinking coffee and eating biscuits. We've got a GP trainee with us tonight. She's a ridiculously young, ridiculously beautiful looking girl who's studying at Imperial College and is here to do a placement as part of her GP rotation. Everyone is clearly trying to impress her. I join them.

One of the older doctors, a short, greying man called Rory, seems to be getting to the end of some long and probably wildly exaggerated story as I pull up a chair. 'She didn't even know she was pregnant!' he ends, triumphantly, as I grab a biscuit. I can guess the beginning of his story. To this day it surprises me that women can last almost nine months without realising that they're going to have a baby. But that's what they always tell us.

'What was the presenting complaint?' I ask.

'Good old indigestion. She'd been to an all-you-can eat Chinese restaurant and reckoned she'd overdone it on the prawn toast or something. It was almost the end of my shift. I was ready for handover and ready to go home. She started screaming in the corridor, waters breaking, contractions thick and fast, the whole nine yards.'

'And you delivered the baby?'

'I certainly did, without so much as a midwife in sight. A baby boy who I'm told weighed in at seven pounds exactly. It was all done and dusted by the time the ambulance arrived. It was bloody noisy, there was a hell of a mess, an awful lot of bleeding and it all got a bit whiffy, to be honest. But other than that it went marvellously well and was text-book smooth.' I could understand my colleague's pride. Delivering babies is a big part of medical training. But I'm sure some of us GPs go our whole careers without putting it into practice. If and when we do then you're guaranteed hero status – especially by the mum. It's all very ER and if you're the right sex they might even name the baby after you. One day – or one night – I'd be over the moon if that happened to me.

Chapter Nine:

Baby Girls and Brave Little Boys

Freddy hasn't been well for quite some time. He was born very early, very small – and as the years passed it turned out that he had very severe Cystic Fibrosis. In the past 18 months alone he has fought so many battles his medical file is probably fatter than he is. He's seven and plenty more battles lie ahead. But tonight it's not him I've been sent to see.

'We're so sorry to call you all the way out here,' his mum says in the hall. 'It's our daughter.' The mum is in her mid-twenties, she's pretty and she's got blond hair and an open, welcoming face. She's also got sad, tired eyes. Once you've seen those you can't help but worry.

'I'm Sue and this is my husband Nathan,' she adds as we walk into the softly lit main bedroom at the front of the house.

'And this is Millie,' he says. He sounds proud, but he too has sad, tired eyes.

The baby girl is wide awake in a soft, comfortable crib. We

normally get parents to bring babies and kids into the base for appointments at night. One very basic reason is that the lights are a lot better there – and Nathan must know this as he flicks on the main light as I approach the cot. 'Sorry baby,' he says as he does so.

'She's just not been feeding or drinking all day. I know it's ridiculous. I know I'm worrying too much. But she had a tough birth and I panicked. I've never done that before,' the mum tells me.

I think I can see her point. The family have probably have had a real challenge getting enough nutrition to their son over the years, because feeding is one of the many challenges of Cystic Fibrosis. In the dead of night they might have transferred the problem to their new daughter.

I run through some quick checks. I want to know the little girl's temperature, I want to see her reactions and how alert she is, I want an idea of her pulse and even her oxygen levels. 'I think little Millie's got a bit of a fever. Nothing serious, just your usual, run of the mill bug. Have you given her anything for it?'

They haven't.

'A bit of paracetemol should bring her temperature down and as soon as she's comfortable she'll feed again,' I conclude. I ask about her fluid intake and check her nappies to see how much is coming out the other end. I'm more than happy with everything I discover. 'If she's not happy in the morning then you could bring her in to see your usual GP. But I think she's going to be just fine.'

'And you think we're panicking parents. You think we're those awful people who dial 999 every time their kids sneeze,' says the mum. This is a different woman to the one who greeted me earlier on. The words have flooded out of her fast. She's right on the edge.

'I don't think that at all. I know how well you cope with your little boy. Everyone has a wobble sometimes. That's what I'm here for. I've got nothing else to do till I clock off at midnight. It's good to get out of the surgery and meet people'

Sue smiles weakly. She gulps a bit. But she seems OK again.

'Do you want to see Freddie? He's slept through all of this,' Nathan says, kindly taking the focus away from his wife. This time there's real pride in his voice.

I follow him across the landing. We creep into what looks like the perfect little boy's room. It's blue, it's got planets and toy planes flying across the ceiling and shelves full of dinosaurs and robots and books along its walls.

'Hello big guy,' I whisper at Freddy's bedside. His pillow and duvet are covered in friendly looking aliens.

'He's been a real hero tonight,' says his dad.

Freddy, far too small for his age, is fast asleep and the picture of contentment.

We creep out and head downstairs. 'Can I get you a hot drink?' a fully recovered Sue asks from the hall. 'The kettle's just boiled,' she adds, seeing my hesitation. I follow her to the kitchen and she makes a round of coffees. She asks me about the other cases I see at nights and the other kids and babies I've seen lately. I ask her about the challenges she's facing as a new mum with a medically challenging older lad.

'She does too much on her own. She doesn't like asking for help,' her husband interrupts at one point.

'It doesn't feel right. We don't like to leave the children with anyone else,' she says. She flashes a quick glance at her husband.

'I don't like to leave the children with anyone else,' she corrects. 'Mollie is our daughter, Freddie is our son. It's our job to look after them.'

There's a bit of a silence. I imagine this battle about care has been going on for some time. I totally respect the little lad's mum. But I hope his dad wins the war. I try to give him some extra firepower by talking through all the respite and specialist services they can access. None of it is new to them and I'm not sure his wife is really listening.

With this final part of my job done I thank them for the coffee, tell them to call if Millie deteriorates, and go back to the car. This proud, exhausted family will muddle on, worrying about their brand new little girl and caring for their vulnerable little boy. I doubt I've done anything that any other GP wouldn't have done tonight. I doubt I've done anything that their family GP wouldn't have done. But I'm glad to have met them and I'm happy to have seen them in their own home. They've reminded me how hard some people work.

Chapter Ten:

A Dog's Life

Doctors and nurses always like chewing the cud and telling stupid stories. One of the GPs we've got on tonight is an older guy called Paul. He's quite a character and can talk for England. Are any of his stories true? I sort of doubt it. But they pass the time if we get a quiet patch in the early hours. Today Paul is on particularly good form. He's one of the old school GPs. Back in the day he'd have turned up at a patient's house in a dinner jacket on New Year's Eve to save a life between his starter and main course. Tonight he's harking back to the 'good old days' yet again. But he's not talking about dinner jackets. He's in the middle of a story about the time he reckons he was called to one of the biggest and roughest council estates in Tottenham, north east London.

The way he tells it, dogs and gangs were roaming the streets – and one particularly fierce pit bull was sitting pawing at the door of the flat he was looking for. When the owner opened the door the dog raced inside and disappeared. Paul reckoned the flat's electricity had been cut off. The only light inside came from a television in the lounge – and judging from the way power cables were passing through a hole punched into the ceiling Paul guessed this was being stolen from the flat next door. 'I was there to check up on a little lad with stomach pains, almost certainly phantom. I had to examine the child in the light from the television,' Paul claimed. 'The whole flat stank. The kid was on a sofa that was damp to the touch. The whole place was freezing and at one point I looked up to see the pit bull squat down and do a massive crap on the hall carpet. I wrote out a prescription and couldn't get out of there fast enough. But the woman stopped me as I headed through the door. "Doctor, you've forgotten your dog," she yelled at me.'

I've got a favourite story of my own about house-calls and dogs. It's about a GP who was supposedly called round to a dog owner who had a stomach ulcer or something. The man was sweating, had vomited blood and was in very bad shape. The doctor starts the examination, records a few facts then gets ready to do a rectal examination. 'I need you to pull your underwear down and lie on your left side while I check inside your back passage,' The GP says. The patient gets in position and closes his eyes firmly as the doctor gloves up and looks for some KY jelly in his bag. At which point the man's dog steps up and starts to give his owner's arse a thorough licking.

'Doctor, is this really necessary?' the patient asks. Or so the story goes.

Tonight I'm spared any such embarrassment. When we start to get busy again I've got a list of house-calls to do. My first is to a 28-year-old man called Antonio who's got renal colic and says his pain levels have gone through the roof. For anyone unfamiliar with the situation, it means a crystallised stone has got stuck in the tube between the kidney and the bladder. It's blocked the pipe and triggered a back-up of urine in the kidney. It also creates waves of pure pain as the muscles try to squeeze the alien invader down and out of the body. Some say it's more painful than getting shot. Some brave men say renal colic hurts more than childbirth – though I doubt they say that to any new mums. Either way it can be a shocker – which is why we used to admit people with it so they can get pain relief in hospital. Nowadays it's fair to say that hospitals have enough to do. If people have bad attacks we try to treat the pain and get sufferers in to see a urologist the following day.

'Have you been sick or felt sick?' I ask once I'm in the man's very minimal, very stylish city flat.

He's not.

'Managing to pass water OK?'

'Yes – but it hurts like hell.'

'No fever?' I ask, checking his temperatures.

He's fine on that score too. I can sort things out so he gets to the urology clinic in daytime hours. Painkillers will have to see him through till then.

'Keep drinking a lot of water, even if it hurts to pee. Walk around a bit as well. And call if it gets worse,' I tell him before heading back to the car and on to the next address.

Chapter Eleven:

House Calls

It's easy to get depressed in the small hours of the morning. There's no fun lying awake at home at 4am and thinking about all your problems. There's no fun gazing out of a portacabin window thinking about society's problems either. But sometimes on a night shift I find myself doing just that. I'm desperate not to turn into a grumpy old man who's at war with the world. But I do get riled about the way some people abuse the system.

Mostly it's due to an incredible sense of entitlement – and a total lack of understanding that someone, somewhere, has to pay for all our GPs, their drivers, their kit and for all the infrastructure that supports them. Sure, we all earn a decent amount as doctors – and some practice-owning GPs earn an absolute fortune. But we pay our taxes on it. Hopefully we pay more into the system than we take out.

Friends of mine in the police force, as well as plenty of hospital and ambulance staff, say there seems to be an ever-widening gap between people who contribute to society and those who take from it or chip away at it. Abuse of the benefit system and abuse of alcohol are our favourite subjects when public service workers get together. I'm sure it's politically incorrect to point the finger at this sort of thing. But if the people on the sharp end of public services can sense it then society – and politicians – should have the guts to examine it.

Sometimes, even after all these years, I have to steel myself to brush off the ingratitude some patients display. There's the sheer, unashamed cheek of some people. There are the ones we speak to on the phone before a visit who ask us to pick up a pizza for them on the way. Or, worse, the ones whose health has been shot by alcohol and who still expect us to collect 'a couple of cans' from the corner shop as we approach. Then there are the ones who expect their out-of-hours GP to take their dog for a quick walk around the block before they leave – or to give them a lift to a friend's house once we've miraculously cured them of whatever they claimed was ailing them.

Every now and then there's that call for everyone using the NHS to get presented with a detailed bill. It would list the total cost of their consultation, their medication and all the other services they've enjoyed. At the end it would say something along the lines of "Amount Due: Zero. Paid in Full by the Great British Taxpayer". Some say this is patronising. Others say the statements might make good citizens feel so guilty about seeing doctors that they miss out on vital care. I can see all sides to the argument. I wish some clever person could square the circle and stop us all from taking too much for granted.

Michael is a case in point. He'd rung his out-of-hours number, spoken to the triage staff and been offered a base appointment with us. That meant he would be seen at a specified time in a place with all the right lighting and equipment to help him. I don't think you can ask for more than that. But Michael had. Apparently he had refused point blank to attend. He probably said it was impossible or had some other manipulative story to hand. I hadn't been asked to speak to him, more's the pity. For whoever had handled the call had taken the easy way out and given in to him. They had caved in and allocated him a house-call. I bet anything that at some point he would have said it was his 'right' to be treated at home. It's not, but by giving in he'll think it is. I'm unusually quiet in the car on the way to his address because I'm in an unusually bad mood. Things don't improve when we get there.

When I stand outside Michael's door he can't hear the bell because his TV is on so loud. It's gone one in the morning. He lives in a flat and he's got neighbours above, below and all around him. I feel bad thumping on the door when he doesn't reply to the bell. He couldn't care less about the noise because everything has to revolve around him. His first questions are about why I've taken so long getting there, why he'd been given so much hassle on the phone when he'd wanted a home visit and when I'm going to give him the painkilling prescription he craves.

'So, Michael, tell me exactly where it hurts.' He had complained about abdominal pain in his initial phone call. That's a useful grey area for people like him. Reporting a bit of pain is always going to get the call handlers' attention, so it has to get everyone else's attention as well. It could just be belly ache. It could be appendicitis. Or it could be a fake.

'All over here,' he says, vaguely pointing around the centre of his stomach. So it's not looking like appendicitis, I think wearily.

'Where exactly? I need you to be more specific if I'm going to help you.'

'Right here then!' he says, suddenly choosing his belly button.

'And what kind of pain is it?'

'What kind of question is that?'

'Is it a constant pain, does it come and go, is it getting better or worse? I'm sure you need help, Michael,' I lie. 'But you have to help me as well.'

Very grudgingly and very unwillingly Michael describes pains that are at once constant and occasional, pains that are dull and pains that are sharp, pains that get worse and pains that never change. I do genuinely listen to him. I do ask the right follow-up questions, I examine him and I try to work out two key things. Is there really something wrong with his belly? And if not, is there some psychological issue that needs to be tackled instead? A few minutes later I conclude that neither case can be proved. At worst, Michael had a bad stomach, the way we all do sometimes. He called us because he could. And now he can't even bring himself to thank me for my time or to apologise for wasting it.

I take a last look around at all the expensive kit in his grubby little flat and try not to rush to any other judgements as I repack my medical bag. I don't feel very good about the world, or about myself, as I show myself out. But I swear I'm not being a complete smug snob here – because I'm the first to agree that the middle classes want just as much bang from their buck.

We really do get urgent, out-of-hours calls from posh families who are off to the Caribbean in the morning and think we'll give their kids some free, last minute travel jabs. A year or so ago an equally posh woman who was due to fly off somewhere fantastic the following day managed to work herself into a full-blown panic attack when she couldn't find her passport. I spent far too long on the phone from the OOH centre talking her down from that one – as well as suggesting a variety of places where the passport might be.

'All sorted, doc?' Roger asks when I get back into the car.

I shrug. 'Bit of a waste of time, really,' I admit. 'Let's see who's next on our list.'

Roger checks the details of our next visit on the computer and releases the handbrake. The street lights are still on, dawn is a while away and the roads are clear. It takes us less than fifteen minutes to get to the address on the screen.

I ring the bell for a top floor flat in a tall, narrow town house. The front door buzzes and I walk past a couple of bikes and a load of junk mail in the hall and head up. A smart, older man comes out on to the top landing to greet me.

'It's my mother. She's 83, she's got dementia but she's never been like this,' he says. 'She's been delirious and irrational before, but she's never been aggressive . Tonight she's been off the scale. She lashed out at the kids – her grandkids. They were terrified, it was awful. She's been shouting, swearing, screaming.'

'The language has been incredible. Words I'd never have expected her to say. It's been like a Jeremy Kyle show. God knows what the neighbours think,' says a slightly younger lady I assume is his wife. She's trying to smile, trying to keep things just a little bit light.

I follow them to see the man's mother. She is not pleased to see me. 'Who the fuck is this?' she screams, her voice as course as her language. 'Get your hands off me you fucking pervert!' she cries. It's hard to imagine that this is the mother of the well-spoken, middle class man at my side. But it's hard to imagine what dementia does, till you see it for yourself. I ignore the anger and the barrage of insults and try not to smile at the lady's son. He's mortified by the whole extraordinary performance.

'Has she moved bedrooms lately or had any other changes to her environment?' I ask. That in itself can trigger agitation in dementia patients.

'No, nothing's changed,' says the son's wife.

'It would be useful to get a urine sample to test for infection,' I begin.

'I've got you one. A very small one,' she says. 'I was a nurse on cruise ships about a hundred years ago. We saw this a lot so I was ready. She had an accident earlier on that made it easier to collect. It smelled bad and it was uncomfortable for her.'

They are useful clues. I take the sample on offer. Testing strips are far more accurate than they used to be. I'll want to get a proper sample to the lab for a definitive analysis. But my gut feeling is that this is a relatively simple urinary tract infection. And the good news is we can sort it out pretty swiftly.

'Will she swallow pills, do you think?' I ask.

Son and daughter-in-law nod. I sort out the medication. The lady glares at me, swears at me but gobbles them down as if they were sweets she's determined not to share. This time I really do let myself smile.

The three of us have a quick chat in the kitchen before I leave. I ought to head straight back to the car but this is the last of my latest block of calls, the family have got some great coffee on the go and I want to hear a bit more about the cruise ship job. When we've talked about that for a few moments I get back to business. I ask if they want me to talk to their kids about their gran's illness but they say they've got it covered.

'It is a struggle, though,' says the son, one of the understatements of the year. 'Even before tonight's little drama it's the weirdness of it that gets to you,' he adds. 'Until tonight she's always been perfectly lucid and utterly normal when she's telling you something. Then she forgets it in a heartbeat. She says the same thing three times in fifteen minutes. Every time you think you've got her, that this is the real her again. But in a moment it's all gone. It's like something shuts down in her brain and takes away everything that's just happened.'

We talk a little about the science of it all and of the research that's going on. We run through everything from hydration to hallucinations. The couple are very clued up and look to have covered most bases already. They've got over one big hurdle, which is to accept that miracle cures aren't really on the cards. The trouble with so many of the afflictions of ageing is that there's not much we can do about them. We age. Our bodies and our brains start to tire and wear out. We're old cars that have been driven into the ground. If our exhaust pipes don't fall off then our fan belts will snap. The trick, I suppose, it to have enough good drives in your day.

I knock back my coffee and feel a bit guilty about Roger out in the car. As I hand back my mug I see a large sliver-framed, black and white photograph on the kitchen dresser. It is of a wildly glamorous looking woman holding a camera. 'Is that your mother?' I ask.

'She was the first female photographer on her local paper in north Wales. Back then it was one of the biggest newspapers of its day,' her son says proudly. 'She moved to London, took pictures of everyone from Churchill to the Beatles. She worked for more than forty years and she travelled the world.' The man smiles and recounts several more of his mum's exploits. It's impossible not to share his pride. The brake fluid and the fuel tank are a bit low. But it sounds as if this lady made the most of her ride.

Chapter Twelve:

Back at Base

The girl is fifteen years old and she's got her dad with her. He does all the talking. The girl, Louise, has had a sore throat and a bad voice, a headache and a rough old cough for five days. On her second day she'd been diagnosed with tonsillitis and her GP had prescribed penicillin. It had been the right thing to do at that point. But apparently the girl's uncle, a drug rep for a pharmaceutical company, hadn't agreed. 'We've been on the phone to him all week and he says penicillin is the worst possible thing to give her. He says it went out years ago. He thinks the doctor should be struck off,' I'm told.

I normally feel sorry for people who are dragged into their relative's medical problems. I never feel sorry for drug reps. Especially when they're wrong. Penicillin might be old but it's still the best treatment for tonsillitis. It should get going in about 24 hours. If it hasn't then something else is going on and we need to try something else – and none of that is penicillin's fault.

'If you can open your mouth wide I'll take a look,' I say to Louise. I don't really need a torch to see that this isn't tonsillitis. A bit of a war is going on in her mouth. Her throat is red and raw and her tonsils are covered in thick white fluid we call exudate. 'That does look nasty. No wonder you're feeling rough,' I say. I ask a few more questions, take a quick look at her eyes and ears then feel her abdomen very gently. A swollen spleen is an indication of glandular fever but I'm very careful when I check tonight. I was out with a bunch of medics on one of my nights off recently and someone had a horror story of squeezing someone's spleen so tight that it ruptured. I doubt that's going to happen here but as it's fresh in my mind I'm not taking any chances.

I turn back to my desk, tap a few details into the computer then move on. I'm pretty sure it is indeed glandular fever – and as I'm on an early shift on hospital premises I reckon we might just be able to get some blood tests done straight away. I send the pair home and tell the girl to rest and stay warm. The labs are open and just over an hour later I ring the family when the test results come through and confirm my diagnosis. It's nice for me to be right – even on something as minor as glandular fever. It's less nice for Louise as she'll be out of commission for some time and will have to take life really slowly as she recovers. If I'm honest, the only annoying thing is the girl's uncle. He was wrong about penicillin but he'll think he was right because his niece has been taken off it. I have a bit of a moan about it with Annie, ignoring the fact that she doesn't really care. Then I get called back to the phones.

Some nights we seem to speak to a lot more worried parents than others. Tonight is one of them. I suppose it's only natural.

There's never a good time to think your baby is unwell. But the middle of the night will always count as one of the worst. Everything seems grim in the isolation of the evening or the early hours of the morning.

So what do parents call about? Nappies can be too wet or too dry. There's a lot of possible fevers and temperatures and little niggles that don't seem to be clearing up. As kids get a little older a lot of things get stuck up noses and in ears. We also get a lot of meningitis calls. Parents panic a lot more in the small hours – and you can hardly blame them. Most of the time the call handlers at NHS Direct or the other OOH firms can talk people through the symptoms and chart the safest course of action. But plenty of calls or call-backs still make it to us – and you have to be careful when they do. Meningitis is a tricky little bugger. You can draw a complete blank looking for signs at midnight only to have your diagnosis totally superseded at dawn.

The good news is that only a tiny minority of house-calls for babies turn into hospital admissions or 999 emergencies. A lot of the time our primary task is just to reassure the parents that everything will be OK in the morning.

And what else takes up a lot of time on the phone? It varies, but some nights it seems as if half the population of my slice of London seems to want – if not necessarily need – a repeat prescription of something or other. Sometimes on a weekend one in four calls can be from people 'needing' a top-up of the contraceptive pill or a new inhaler for their asthma. If they really do need it we try to sort things out with a late night pharmacist. If we need extra detail we'll get them to come to us. A house-call because you've run out of the pill? You can ask. I don't think you're going to get. A house-call because you've got a bad rash and are embarrassed to be seen out in public? Sorry, again, but it's a 'no' from me.

Tonight my fellow GP Anil takes over on the phones just after midnight and I head into my surgery to see some appointments. The first is a twenty-two year-old man who's been asked to come in several mornings after the night before.

He was clearly involved in some sort of scrap. He's got lacerations to his forehead and the side of his face. There's extensive bruising and a tasty black eye is developing.

'I was out on the town,' he begins when I ask for the background. 'I got hit or I fell over or someone hit me or something else happened. I don't know what.'

'So you'd been drinking?'

'I was out of it that night. I just dunno what happened.'

'And this was three nights ago?'

'Yeah.'

I ask more questions but don't get many more answers. He's not sure if he lost consciousness but he's not had any nausea or vomiting. As he didn't lose his phone or any cash he doesn't think he was mugged and he didn't call the police or go to hospital at the time. He just woke up, on his girlfriend's sofa, looking like he'd been in a plane crash. I take a closer look at his war wounds, check his motor responses and eye movements. His vision is good and while his eye socket is tender there's no obvious injury to the eye itself. His bite seems fine and he has no problems opening or closing his mouth.

'So there's no other pain or new pain that's made you come here tonight?' I ask.

'My girlfriend asked around at work and someone said I might have brain damage.'

'Because of the accident, right?' I say, judging that he's got a sense of humour.

'Very funny. Yes, because of the accident.'

'Well I think you'd know about it if things were serious. But as you've come all the way in here you might as well get yourself checked out at A&E. If you did lose consciousness then we ought to take a proper look. They can do some x-rays and a scan. I'll give you a print-out to hand in at the front desk when you get there.'

I tap his details into the computer then briefly turn into the guy's dad by telling him it's a bad idea to drink so much, you don't know what you're doing. Or to have friends who don't stick around when you need them most.

'You'll take a bit more care on your next night out?' I ask, as he stands up to leave.

'Yes doctor,' he lies.

Chapter Thirteen:

Calling 999

I'm not sure if it's true but from the seventies onwards everyone had high hopes when all our Casualty departments started to rebrand themselves as A&E. The thinking was clear. Casualty sounded too welcoming. It sounded as if it encompassed far too many conditions that could easily wait till the morning. But Accident and Emergency? You only go if you've been in an accident or if it's an emergency. Surely you can't get much clearer than that? The powers that be were convinced that as soon as the new phrase got stuck in the national consciousness then all the frivolous admissions would stop. It hasn't quite worked out like that. Today A&E has more frivolous visits than ever. People try to use it as a walk-in health centre. They try to use it for on-demand care and easy second opinions. They abuse it, to be frank.

Do patients abuse the out-of-hours service as well? Some do. The kind of people who come in to one of our bases at ten at night, two in the morning or at any point over the weekend will depend, to a large extent, on who takes the initial call and who follows it up. Call centre staff who don't sit with the doctors and nurses are probably a bit more appointment happy – though there are all sorts of rumours of bonuses awarded or withdrawn at some centralised OOH operations based on the number of callers who can be fobbed off onto A&E. When we're answering calls in-house at one of the smaller set-ups we genuinely try to base it on perceived clinical need. Over the years I've had people come in for all sorts of reason. People get an appointment because they've got the tip of a cotton bud stuck in their ear – even though there's no sign of it when we take a look. They call up about lots of flu-like symptoms and can come in to display all sorts of rashes. We see people with burns that aren't healing, sore fingers, frozen shoulders, giddy spells, persistent coughs, green phlegm, black stools, high temperatures, sports injuries; you name it we hear about it. People walk into doors, hit their heads on low shelves, get drunk and forget to take important medication. We see them with allergic reactions, pimply tongues, swollen eyes, thick ears – and almost anything else you can imagine. A lot of the time we know exactly what to do because the infections, illnesses and injuries are clear cut. Others are a little more mysterious.

'House-call over in Clapham if you're free?' says Roger from my office door after I'd cleared a long backlog of the former cases.

'I'll see you in the car.'

We talk about his daughter's latest half marathon on the drive and Roger extracts yet another £25 from me in sponsorship.

Roger is grinning away and celebrating his financial victory when he double parks outside a big, semi-detached family house on a narrow leafy street. No-one's grinning inside. There's a distinctly odd atmosphere. For some reason I sense that the house is fully occupied. But only one person greets and speaks to me. He's a distant, distracted-looking man. He's of Bangladeshi origin and looks to be in his early thirties.

'You're not from our surgery, are you? You're a locum, right?' he says as he leads me up the stairs.

'I'm a doctor from the out-of-hours service,' I say. I don't really like the world locum.

'You're not based in the surgery?'

'No I'm not. Why do you ask?'

'No reason.'

He leads me into a bedroom on the first floor and I start to guess the reason why. A very sick elderly man is lying back in bed. A very sick elderly man whose skin is a lifeless, yellowy hue and who seems to have a very distinctive shape. He flashes me a weak glance. The whites of his eyes are anything but. I can't pre-judge, but I think I know exactly what's wrong with him. The big issue is how bad it has become – and how fast we have to act.

'What's been the problem tonight?' I ask, trying to keep things as business like as possible.

'He's in pain. His stomach is not good. I think he's bleeding. His English isn't great. I can translate anything.'

I lean towards the patient and begin my examination. A lot of air freshener has been thrown around this room. It looks as if toothpaste has been put inside the man's mouth. But none of it can hide the smell of booze. The man looks at me then he looks around the room though he doesn't seem to know why. 'I'm going to take a look at his chest and abdomen,' I say. I lift the sheets. The man's son opens his dad's pyjamas. More clues hit me all the time. The man's chest is hairless. It may have been like that all his life. Or it could be another key sign of cirrhosis caused by a lifetime of drinking. It's ironic, but tough men who drink all their lives can see their testosterone levels plummet. They can lose all their body hair. They can even develop breasts – a key detail left out of most alcohol advertising campaigns.

'I'm going to tap your chest in a few places,' I tell the man. His son repeats it and I begin. I listen as I move my hands around. The sounds change, just as I expected. I ask the man to move on to his side and tap a little more.

'You think he's bleeding? From his back passage?' I ask.

The son nods. I take a look but my diagnosis is already done and my decision is made. 'Your father is being cared for, where?' I ask, taking off my gloves and getting my phone out of my bag.

The son looks away. 'We care for him at home.'

'But he's been getting care? He'll be getting treatment somewhere?'

The man looks away again. And this, I know, is why the man is different to almost every other patient we have at night. This man doesn't want his usual family GP to come out and see him. He specifically wants an anonymous locum to visit in the middle of the night. If your culture or religion says you can't drink alcohol then I imagine you want as few people as possible to know that you're dying of cirrhosis. This weak, elderly man may have been taken to A&E or walk-in centres every now and then. The family may be hoping to top things up with a bit of out-of-hours care like this. The thinking must be that what happens at night stays at night – what happens in random, out-of-area hospitals stays there as well. It's time to disillusion them.

'Your father has to go to hospital tonight. I'll make the call for you.'

There's a long, awkward pause. The natural thing, if you waste time asking questions at all, is to ask about the condition and the prognosis. Tonight I'm asked just one question. 'Will our GP be told?'

'He will. We're long past the point where this can be hidden,' I say. 'I'll arrange an ambulance. Your father will probably be admitted to Kings where he'll get great care. The care he should have been having for some time.'

The man does, at last, look abashed. 'It's been complicated,' he says haltingly.

I put up my hand. 'It doesn't matter now. Let's just get your dad to hospital.'

I call 999 and explain the situation to the operator. When I hang up the son does finally pepper me with questions about the diagnosis and his dad's prospects. The blue lights swing through the front room a little while later. The crew scoop the man on to a trolley and wheel him out of the house.

'If he dies, what will he die of?' the son asks, his final question before joining his dad in the ambulance.

I'm pretty sure he wants me to come up with a culturally neutral answer like pneumonia. I'm not going to do it.

'We should focus on getting your father through the next few days,' I say. The battle over cause of death, when it comes, will be for someone else.

Chapter Fourteen:

My Thoughts on Death

Her face is calm and soft. Her body is relaxed and comfortable. She was seventy six and she had died in bed. There is no sign of trauma, no sign of pain. Instead there is an overwhelming air of peace about her. Not so her husband. He's in shock. He's broken. He can't yet grieve because all he feels is guilt.

'I wasn't there,' he says, again and again. He stands up tall in front of me. He pulls himself up as straight as his spine will allow. He's in dirty, gardening clothes but it's as if he's on parade. This poor, broken man could be in the dock. He's acting as if I'm his judge. 'I was at the allotment. I go every afternoon. I've always gone every afternoon. I don't come home till gone eight in the summer. So I wasn't here for her. I wasn't here when she needed me.'

'Mr Lamb shall we sit down? Shall we go into the living room for a moment?'

'I won't leave her again, sir,' he tells me. He's a good forty years older than me.

'Then let's sit here. Please sit down Mr Lamb.'

This stiff, stunned gentleman does, finally, unbend and sits on the very edge of the chair by his late wife's bed.

'I wasn't there, sir' he says again. His voice is deeper now, it's trembling and his breath is catching in his throat. His eyes look into nowhere, possibly into the past. Sadness and even shame at his absence are written all over his tired, weather beaten face. Regret hangs so very heavy in the air.

I look at him and wonder if I should tell him something. It might be too complicated and it might not make sense. It might not even be right. But it's a theory of mine, something that few people say but lots of doctors believe. It's that some people want to die alone. Some people choose to.

I got an inkling of this many years ago when I was working in a hospital in the Midlands as part of my training. I saw so many families sitting around so many beds. The patients they loved were barely or rarely conscious. But no-one ever wanted to leave the ward or the room. Along with all the other staff, I watched as families and friends set up rotas and organised their lives so there was always someone there for the person they loved.

And then, more often than you'd think, I saw that the final moment came when the person on watch had gone to the loo, for a coffee or a cigarette or for an update from one of the doctors or nurses.

'I wasn't there,' we heard again and again.

But I like to think that the patient wanted it that way. Dignity is important to all of us. We are all proud, in our own way. Do we like being powerless and impotent, lying in a bed while so many people loom over us and watch our every breath? Doctors are used to death, but I still think about it all the time. Not everyone wants to take that final step while the ones they love are with them. We don't know what will happen. We don't want to upset the ones we love. So we hold on for them. That's what they're telling us to do. That's what they want us to do.

So imagine, for a moment, the relief when the room is silent. When the watching eyes have gone. When we're alone and we feel we've regained a brief moment of control. That's the moment we can relax, we can let go and we can rest. It can be the moment when we choose to die.

Will this untested, unlikely theory of mine be any comfort to the broken Mr Lamb tonight? I don't know. I don't know if he'll hear me, even if I try to articulate it to him. Instead I fall back on the few lines that I know will help. 'She wouldn't have felt any pain,' I say quietly but firmly. 'Mr Lamb, your wife was at peace.'

Chapter Fifteen:

A Quiet Patch

One more night shift then I'm off to Canada for a three week holiday. A group of us are flying to Vancouver, going sailing, fishing, camping and then, I hope, going drinking. One more night to go – and it's starting off in very good humour.

One of my colleagues has just come back from a call to a man in a tiny bedsit whose supposedly extreme bellyache was cured, just as she leaned in close to examine him, by a very long, very loud trump. The rest of us try not to laugh as we hit the phones, trying to meet our targets and return urgent calls within twenty minutes and other calls within sixty.

A few other funny stories get thrown around as the hours go by. And there is a lot of material on the night shift. Everyone seems to think it's the A&E doctors who get the laughs when people turn up with vegetables, shampoo bottles or other odd objects stuck where the sun doesn't shine – and start to spin a fantastic variety of improbable stories about how the unfortunate incident occurred.

In reality I reckon we see and hear just as many of those stories. If you're a middle-aged pillar of the community and you've wedged some kitchen implement up your back passage do you really want to head on over to A&E – especially if sitting down to drive might be just a little bit uncomfortable? Do you want to shuffle into a crowded waiting area and stand in line at the reception desk? Do you want to speak to a nurse behind a reinforced safety screen who can't really hear above the chaos of an inner city night? 'Sorry, you've got what? A pepper mill? You're going to have to speak up, sir. The pepper mill is stuck where? Sorry can you repeat that? I need to type in the information now for when you're seen.'

And do you really want to be there in one of those split seconds when the room goes unaccountably quiet and the receptionist stops typing and looks you right in the eye. 'You've stuck a pepper mill up your arse? And your name, sir?'

Not that this will be the end of it. Your next challenge is to edge back to the waiting area, knowing that every English speaker in the room is watching to see whether you choose to sit or stand while you wait. And do you want to risk seeing someone you know avert their gaze as they snigger and pretend to read yesterday's Metro?

No, far better to hide behind a telephone, call an out-of-hours number and get one of us to come to see you at home. It's still going to be embarrassing. Your usual GP will be sent the case details in the morning. But at least you won't have to face him for a while. And when you do you can deny all knowledge and say it was mistaken identity. You can move house or change your name if you're really upset. I'm sure people do.

Tonight my first two home visits are relatively routine. The last one is more memorable but it's very far from funny. Sadly it's very typical. It's mental health.

Chapter Sixteen:

Talking Him Down

'His name is Eddie and he's lived across there for about five years. There are problems all the time. If it gets bad we've been told who to call and when. Good luck, you're going to need it.'

With that, the man closes his front door, and, I assume, goes back to bed. I step across to the front door of the flat opposite.

I knock, wait, ring the buzzer, wait, then test the door. It doesn't open. I knock again – and it opens fast. A man is standing there. He's in his early thirties, probably a little younger than me. He's naked, he's probably incontinent and he's almost entirely covered in faeces. He flashes me a brilliant smile, then he darts down the hall. I follow him with a heavy heart. The flat is warm and the smell is quite shocking. Patches of carpet squelch under my shoes.

'I'm going to jump out of the window! I'm going to jump out of the window!' the man tells me from the living room. There is joy, pure jubilation on his face. I flash a quick look at the window behind him. It looks to be made up of those square, pull-in panels. I'll check in a minute, but I think they pivot on their base and I doubt they open more than a few inches up top. Even if they did I'm not sure this man would fit through. Genuine threats of suicide need decisive action. But they are less common than you'd think. And this isn't one of them.

'Eddie, my friend, can you stand still just for a moment. Stand so I can take a look at you and make sure you've not hurt yourself somehow.'

Eddie isn't keen on standing still. He's not keen on standing at all any more. He crumples on to the ground and curls up a little. I bend down and approach him slowly to keep everything as unthreatening as possible. He decides to growl a bit as I edge around him to see if there are any wounds or deformities under the faeces. He laughs when I stand up slowly to check the window latches.

'I can fly out of there. I can fly and you can't stop me,' he crows.

I give him a non-committal smile. I want to keep a lid on everything, to keep everything as low-key as possible for as long as possible. Overall I'm pretty sure I could have this man admitted to psychiatric hospital. I could have him sectioned. But what a nightmare for the ambulance staff who'll have to get him there and all the people who'll have to admit him. All the other agencies and the local mental health crisis team will have to get involved too, probably using people like me who've never met the man before, haven't got his trust and don't know all his idiosyncrasies and triggers. The whole thing could set the guy back on whatever road he's travelling. It would cost a fortune as well. All for someone who has no real intention of self-harm and can probably be calmed down till tomorrow.

At that point his usual social workers, case workers and his regular GP can take over. He'll have a case file that could fill a small bookshop. These people will know him. They've clearly briefed his neighbours pretty well. They've probably sorted out his windows. With a bit of luck he might even trust them.

'Eddie, mate, you must be freezing down there. Why don't we get you in the bathroom? Just for a minute so you can sit under the shower. It'll be warm. It's all good. Let's find the bathroom pal.'

Eddie isn't keen on that idea either. He's a big guy, about six-foot two and while he's got wild hair and a filthy beard he's built like a soldier. One of the other GPs we've got on tonight is a tiny, newly qualified woman called Nina. I wouldn't fancy her chances with this guy. I don't really fancy mine.

'Look at that window. I'm jumping out of it. I'm flying forever. I'll show you how to fly.'

'Eddie, if you're going to fly then let's clean up first, right? It's cold out there too. You'll want some clothes on, buddy. Come on, let's get you sorted.'

The shower isn't entirely successful to be honest. Eddie sits down and has a bit of a weep before cheering up, grabbing the shower head and spraying me with water. I draw a bit of a blank on the clean clothes front as well. But any clothes are better than nothing at this stage. A whole world of bin bags are piled high in his small, smelly, black-walled bedroom. I open the first of them gingerly but don't find any hidden horrors. I find him something relatively fresh to wear and I persuade him to give it a try.

By the time he's dressed he's forgotten all about flying out of the window. If he'd stayed on the edge I could have sedated him to see him through the night. But that could have caused problems in the morning. Psychiatrists won't do mental state examinations when people are on those kinds of medication. So the man's care could hit another speed bump till his next assessment takes place. All in all I reckon it's best to leave this sleeping dog to lie. Talking therapy really can work wonders. It won't change Eddie's world or redirect his future. If this exact same incident happened again I could use exactly the same words and actions and get an entirely different response. Next time he may have to leave his flat. But tonight he can stay.

'Do you want to try cleaning up a bit?' I ask after a while.

He does, luckily enough. We clean about five per cent of the affected surface area of his home then Eddie tells me he's tired. He doesn't say another word to me. He turns tail, goes to his bedroom, gets into bed and closes his eyes. I lean closer. He's sucking his thumb and he's asleep, within seconds of his head hitting the pillow. I carry on listening to his breathing. If he's faking it then he's a very good actor, which I doubt. Lucky sod, I think to myself. I wish I could sleep that well.

I leave him be, do a quick hazard check round the flat and hope whoever cleans for him has nerves of steel. I leave a note for his neighbour thanking them for calling us and saying Eddie is calm and I'll be setting up appointments so he is seen by the professionals in the morning.

Back at base I put Eddie's care wheels in motion and crack on with the list of call-backs that have built up for me. It's a funny period, the last few hours of the morning shift. London's surgeries will be opening soon. If something happens now and can't wait till eight o'clock then it's probably a job for A&E. Sometimes we're still out on house-calls and we don't get back till gone clocking-off time. But if we're at our base we're normally quite chilled. These are the times when you think you've got the best job in medicine.

Just before 8am I take a last look at breakfast TV in the waiting area then head back to my room to log off my computer and lock away my medical kit. I say goodbye to the team. Then I head out into the morning rush hour. I love that feeling – seeing hundreds of other people preparing to start the working day and knowing that mine is well and truly over.

When I get home I'm going to put my dirty clothes in the wash then have a bit of a sleep before I pack for Canada. At least I won't get jet lag on the trip. Working nights means your body clock is so messed up at the best of times that you could circumnavigate the globe and not feel that different to normal.

I've not yet booked a single shift for my return. Even in London, out-of-hours doctors always seem to be in demand so there's no real need. And I might take a break from nights anyway. I might do some day shifts or I might try a bit of prison or armed forces medicine. I could follow one of my doctor friends and do holiday repatriation or even cruise-ship medicine. That's the great thing about being a doctor – you've always got options. Maybe one day, if I stumble across the right surgery, I might even settle down and apply for a permanent job. Maybe one day.